Limitless

Master The Art Of Memory Improvement With Brain Training To Learn Faster, Remember More, Increase Productivity And Improve Memory

trustgenics

Copyright Notice

No part of this book may be reproduced or transmitted in any form whatsoever, electronic, or mechanical, including photocopying, recording, or by any information storage or retrieval system without expressed written, dated and signed permission from the author. All copyrights are reserved.

Disclaimer

Reasonable care has been taken to ensure that the information presented in this book is accurate. However, the reader should understand that the information provided does not constitute legal, medical or professional advice of any kind.

No Liability: this product is supplied "as is" and without warranties. All warranties, express or implied, are hereby disclaimed. Use of this product constitutes acceptance of the "No Liability" policy. If you do not agree with this policy, you are not permitted to use or distribute this product.

We shall not be liable for any losses or damages whatsoever (including, without limitation, consequential loss or damage) directly or indirectly arising from the use of this product.

Claim your FREE Audiobook Now

The Confident New You - Develop Your Confidence and Start Living the Life You Deserve

Do you get lost for words around other people, or do you suffer from social anxiety? Are you more concerned about how you look to other people?

If your confidence is always holding you back from achieving what you really want in your life, or if you have always been super shy with no confidence then read on.

You're about to discover how to be confident in any situation. Find out how to make a great first impression and keep the conversation going, without appearing awkward.

Learn to stop thinking negatively about yourself and conquer your fears to gain unstoppable confidence at anything. Even if you don't have low confidence, you can always benefit from improved confidence - there are always greater heights to reach.

THE CONFIDENT NEW YOU

DEVELOP YOUR CONFIDENCE AND START LIVING THE LIFE YOU DESERVE

DARCY CARTER

Trustgenics

Master key ideas in math, science, and computer science through problem solving.

Sign up for Free Now

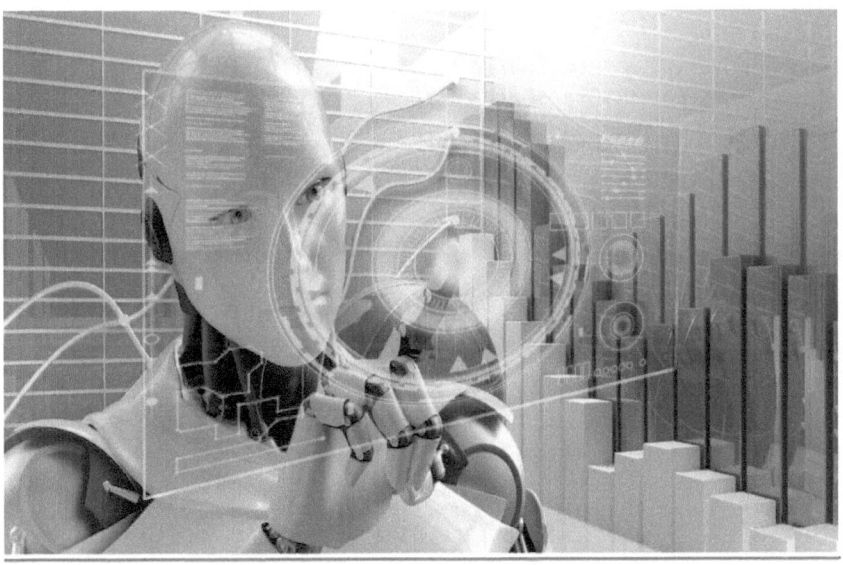

Table Of Contents

Introduction

Chapter 1: Impress People with Expert Level Memory Recall

Chapter 2: Negative Effects on Your Brain Explained, Including Fatigue, Nutrition, and Hormones

Chapter 3: Apply Memorization Techniques to All Areas of Your Personal and Professional Life. Remember Names, Numbers, Lists, and Even Impress Your Friends

Chapter 4: By Memorizing a Pack of Playing Cards

Chapter 5: Discover the Secret of the Oldest Memory Trick that Dates Back to Around 500 B.C.

Chapter 6: Powerful Memory Techniques and Memory Skills to Increase Brain Function

Chapter 7: Protect Your Memory from Deteriorating Due to the Aging Process

Conclusion

Introduction

Surely, you have had instances when you forgot where you placed your keys, your doctor's appointment, important deadlines with clients, and even your wedding anniversary. You may have seen people and struggled to recall their names even though you remembered their faces.

Well, you are not alone. Millions of people all over the world experience the same thing. Just like you, they also blank out and forget stuff.

However, there really is no such thing as "bad memory". People forget things because they do not use their memories to the fullest extent.

Scientists have determined that the human brain is able to adapt and change in such a staggering manner – regardless of a person's age. This brain capability is better referred to as neuroplasticity. The human brain has the great ability to alter present connection, form new neural connections, and react and adapt in constantly changing means. All this can be achieved once the proper stimuli is applied.

Whether you are a student studying for the final exams, a working professional interested in sharpening your memory, or an elderly person looking to preserve and enhance the gray matter in your brain as you age, you can use a lot of strategies to improve your memory and mental performance.

A powerful memory can help you succeed in school, at work, and in life. It can help you learn faster as well as give you more opportunities to earn more money.

Even if becoming a memory master is not your main goal, brain training will surely be beneficial for you.

So, if you want to improve your memory, start reading the following chapters.

Thanks for downloading this book. I hope you enjoy it!

Chapter 1: Impress People with Expert Level Memory Recall

Memrise founder and CEO Ed Cooke said that attending business school or getting a consultant is important in business. You can succeed on your own merits. In fact, Cooke spent most of his 20s joining and winning competitions. He used to memorize the order of sixteen decks of cards, for instance.

His experience is the perfect preparation for his role. After all, Memrise is an effective tool that helps individuals learn anything, from foreign languages to scientific facts. It involves the use of fun associations to make ideas or words stick. Later in this book, you will learn more about the strategies that they use to sharpen memory.

Likewise, Malcolm Gladwell brought up the theory of deliberate practice in his book entitled Outliers. This proves that excellence does not always have to come from talent, but rather devotion and hard work. If you spend thousands of hours on deliberate practice, you can develop a skill.

As the saying goes, "practice makes perfect". For example, typing may seem like a simple skill. You type words on your computer without even looking at your keyboard. You have already mastered the placement of the letters, numbers, and special characters.

However, you have not always been this good, right? When you first started to use a computer, you had a hard time typing because you did not know the placement of characters yet. As time goes by, you get better at typing. You get used to the activity because you keep doing it over and over.

So, what makes practice deliberate?

Well, there are certain characteristics that you have to watch for.

For starters, it has to require effort. Otherwise, everybody will do it and it will not separate average individuals from world class performers anymore.

It must be designed to enhance performance. It has to prompt you to push your limits and get out of your comfort zone. You have to do something that you do not understand and have never done before.

You have to repeat doing it until you nail it. Self-mastery is crucial. There should come a time when doing it becomes effortless, natural, and automatic because you are so used to doing it.

Moreover, it has to have feedback. You should be able to tell whether or not you are doing it correctly. This way, you can improve your ways in case it is necessary.

Daniel Coyle, author of The Talent Code, recommends choosing a target and reaching for it. Then, you should assess the gap between your reach and your target before going back to the first step.

Automatic Plateaus

Some people wonder why they need a form of practice that is different from a normal one. The answer to this is that performance plateaus are necessary for improvement and growth.

For example, a man may drive his whole life, but never develop the skills of a race car driver. After learning how to drive, his performance has plateaued and his skill level became stagnant.

In general, developing a skill requires full attention and effort. Eventually, the task or activity becomes automatic if you render enough hours in doing it. During this time, further improvement and performance plateaus should be aimed for.

Breaking Down Skills

In order for you to do an impossible task, you have to break it down into smaller possible tasks.

To deliberately practice, you have to break down one skill into smaller parts, each of which should be practiced. Repeat doing these parts until they become automatic. Then, you have to work on them further in order to attain refinement. Only then will you be able to say that you have mastered the skill.

For example, if you want to learn programming, you need to have certain sub-skills, such as familiarity with control structures and general computer literacy. You have to learn these basic skills before you can move on to intermediate ones, and consequently to advanced.

Before you can create an application, you have to be familiar with how stack works. You have to learn about the command line, as well as know how to use the Internet. Before you can be good at speed reading, you have to have a wide vocabulary. You have to understand what you are reading so that you can quickly move on to new chapters.

This is true for all skills, no matter how mundane they may seem. You have to master the most basic part before you can move to a higher level. Everything, from writing to solving math problems to playing a musical instrument, requires consistent practice.

Neutral Configuration and Paying Attention

Ralph Waldo Emerson once said that a man becomes whatever he always thinks about.

There is a connection between attention and neural reconfiguration. The theory behind it is that the brain wires anything that you focus on. When you lean on neural structure often, it grows further.

Consider mindless practicing, for example. When you sit down with an instrument or run through a song haphazardly, nothing sticks. On the other hand, if you focus as you play through a song, every note sticks. You remember everything. There is a scientific reason behind this.

Attention makes your brain grow. When you focus on something, it sticks with you for a long time.

How can your attention improve?

There are a variety of ways on how to improve attention, including stimulants such as nicotine, Adderall, and caffeine. You can also pay attention to attention, particularly by practicing Vipassana meditation.

You can also eliminate distraction. For example, you can turn off your phone or TV. If you tend to overthink or be anxious over certain things, you can set a specific time for it. Allot a worry period each day. This way, you can think about the things that bother you for a short while and spend the rest of your day doing important tasks.

Insight, Recognition, and Memory

World-class athletes and performers got to where they are today through consistent practice. They trained day and night, wasting no opportunity to improve their skill.

Anna-Maria Botsari simultaneously played 1102 chess matches in 2001 and won 1095 times. Marc Lang simultaneously played blindfold chess and won nineteen times.

You may think that memorizing board positions is easy for chess players and that it is in their nature. However, this is not the case. These individuals practiced for years. They developed their long-term working memory after many years of training.

The earliest proof for this can be found in de Groot's study of chess recall. He worked with skilled chess players and told them to recall various board positions. The participants did well when showed actual board positions. They did poorly when shown random board positions.

This study was then replicated a few more times in bridge, chess, dance, field hockey, figure skating, basketball, physics, computer programming, music, and electronics.

The theory behind this is that untrained individuals can hold around seven numbers in their short-term memory at once. Short-term memory is generally limited, but you may get around it through chunking.

For example, if you are given meaningful board positions, you may hold bigger chunks in your memory. When you read, you hold words in your memory instead of letters.

This is the way expert memory functions. Humans essentially have a glue function that occurs during practice. According to Herbert Simon, a chunk takes around thirty seconds of focused attention to materialize. A person of expert level has already created fifty thousand to nearly two million chunks. This is equivalent to four hours of practice each day for a decade.

Intuition

Intuition usually distinguishes experts. Take the blitz style in chess, for example. Generally, it works that every side is given five minutes on the clock as well as ten seconds for every turn. Based on the conditions, a person should rely on his intuition instead of thought.

It is not surprising that great chess players easily beat weak ones during blitz matches. Why does this happen? Where does intuition come from? The answer to this question is long-term memory.

You see, when your brain makes a chunk, it gets saved in the long-term memory. So, a chess master has already created thousands of chunks from his previous matches. He already knows which moves should be taken and which ones should not.

Intuition is when the brain recalls something it has already seen before and then matches the patterns that it sees in the present. So, when a chess player views the board, his long-term memory retrieves information that can be helpful. He remembers strong moves and similar positions. This allows him to take the right move.

Insight is the effortless and fast recall of cached experiences. Rather than compute something multiple times, you can simply retrieve it from your memory.

The human brain works the same way. When you encounter a problem or experience, you use effortful computation to deal with it. This is then chunked and saved in your long-term memory. When you encounter a similar problem in the future, you can use look ups to solve it.

The Mental Molasses Hypothesis

A single neuron can fire one to two hundred times per second. This is basically akin to a processor's clock speed in which every neuron is a processor. Brain neurons operate at a maximum speed of 200 hertz while a processor can reach speeds of 4 billion hertz or 4 gigahertz. This only shows that a central processing unit is actually twenty million times faster than a neuron.

So, where does the difference lie between the two? Well, a modern central processing unit may have four to eight processors, but the human brain has one hundred billion neurons. Hence, it can be regarded as a parallel processor.

Then again, the brain cannot compute answers to problems. It can only retrieve answers from memory. The human brain is a massive cache. It can compute, but it is slow. Thoughts are retrieved from long-term memory. Even in a conversation, you may notice that you are merely repeating things that you have heard or thought in the past.

In Conclusion

Humans are basically memory machines. Expertise is merely a result of how much chunks or specific knowledge has been stored in memory. Such chunks are made during deliberate practice, which requires intense focus. In turn, intense focus is required to produce neural reconfiguration.

So, how can you apply this to everyday life? You can use Anki to boost your chunk production. You can take a skill that you want to improve and break it down. Determine any weakness that you have and create an elaborate plan to improve the skill. See to it that you break this plan into smaller chunks so that you do not get intimidated or overwhelmed.

When you are done creating your plan, you should use the Pomodoro technique every day. Only focus on deliberate practice. Refrain from letting any distraction get the best of you. Refresh your mind and body through meditation and a good diet. See to it that you also review your plan and training periodically to ensure that everything is on point. Eliminate anything that does not work. Do not be afraid to get out of your comfort zone to try something new.

Chapter 2: Negative Effects on Your Brain Explained, Including Fatigue, Nutrition, and Hormones

Fatigue, poor nutrition, hormonal imbalances, and stress can all have negative effects on you. These factors can cloud your mind and cause you to perform poorly.

How Fatigue and Stress Negatively Affect the Brain

Fatigue can make it difficult for you to focus and manage your moods. It can even cause you to have mental block, irritability, and lack of motivation. When you are stressed out and fatigued, it can really be hard to do anything properly.

Stress, in particular, is bad for both the body and mind. It can cause unpleasant physical symptoms such as chest pain and headaches as well as mood issues such as sadness and anxiety. It can also cause behavioral problems such as overeating and anger outbursts.

Even worse, stress can have a serious impact on the brain. Whenever you are stressed, your brain experiences multiple reactions that are naturally designed to protect itself against possible threats. There are times when stress is necessary, such as when it helps you remember details. For the most part, however, stress is not good for you.

According to researchers, stress can shrink the brain's volume and contribute to mental health problems.

Chronic stress causes mental illness.

A study published in Molecular Psychiatry has shown that chronic stress can cause long-term brain changes, which in turn can make you prone to anxiety and mood disorders. Likewise, stress can cause mental and emotional disorders, including depression.

At the University of California in Berkeley, researchers conducted several experiments to look at the effects of chronic stress on the human brain. They have found that stress leads to the production of myelin-producing cells with abnormally low neuron count.

This occurs when the myelin in the brain becomes excessive and starts to interfere with the balance and timing of communication. The researchers also found that stress also negatively affects the hippocampus of the brain.

Stress changes the structure of the brain.

This is perhaps one of the most shocking effects of stress. Researchers have found that chronic stress can cause long-term changes in the function and structure of the brain.

As you know, your brain consists of gray matter and neurons. These support cells are responsible for problem-solving and decision-making. Your brain also has white matter, which consists of axons that are linked to the other areas of the brain. It is called white matter because of the myelin or the fatty, white sheath that surrounds the axons. These axons speed up electrical signals to allow information to be communicated to the brain.

When myelin is overproduced because of chronic stress, the structure of the brain can change and the gray and white matter can have an imbalance. According to researchers, those who suffer from post-traumatic stress disorder also tend to have gray and white matter imbalances as well as other brain abnormalities.

Daniela Kaufer, a researcher and psychologist, stated that stress does not always affect the neural networks and the brain in a similar manner. The positive type of stress can help people do well in the event of an emergency or challenge. Their brains can be wired positively, causing them to be more productive and resilient.

On the contrary, chronic stress only yields problems. So, stress either improves you or destroys you. It can either make you resilient or prone to mental illnesses, depending on the white matter pattern you have.

Stress causes brain cells to die.

Researchers at the Rosalind Franklin University of Medicine and Science have found that a socially-stress event can kill the new neurons inside the hippocampus of the brain.

The hippocampus is the area of your brain that is associated with learning, memory, and emotions. It is also where new brain cell formation or neurogenesis takes place.

The researchers used rats in their experiments. In one cage, they let two old rats mix with young rats for twenty minutes. The young rats experienced aggression from the older rats.

When the researchers examined the rats, they discovered that the young rats that experienced aggression had six times higher levels of cortisol than the ones that did not experience aggression.

Furthermore, even though both groups of young rats had the same amount of new neurons, the ones that experienced stress had a reduction of nerve cells. Thus, although stress may not affect the formation of new neurons, it can still affect their survival.

Stress causes the brain to shrink.

Anyone, regardless of health condition, can experience brain shrinkage if they are exposed to stress. In particular, the areas of their brain that is connected to memory, emotions, and metabolism will be affected.

According to researchers, the stress that you experience on a daily basis can accumulate over time and eventually result in mental illnesses. You may not notice the effects of chronic daily stress right away, but they can actually make your brain shrink when you get exposed to traumatic and intense stressors.

Researchers at Yale University conducted a study that involved one hundred healthy individuals. These participants gave information about the stressful encounters they have had in life.

The researchers found that being exposed to stress, no matter how much time has passed, caused the gray matter in the participants' prefrontal cortex to shrink. The prefrontal cortex is the area of your brain that is associated with emotions and self-control.

So, if you are constantly exposed to stressful situations, you can have a harder time dealing with stress in the future. This is especially true if you have to have integrated social processing, effortful control, or emotion regulation.

Stress negatively affects memory.

When you are stressed, you may have a difficult time remembering events and important details. Even mild stress can negatively affect your memory. For example, you may struggle to recall where you placed your car keys or your briefcase.

In 2012, researchers have found that chronic stress negatively affects spatial memory. This is your ability to remember details associated with location and spatial orientation. In 2014, another study has shown that high cortisol levels can cause short-term memory to decline.

In essence, stress can either help or hurt your memory. For instance, timing is among the variables that cause stress to affect memory. According to researchers, if stress is experienced immediately prior to learning, memory consolidation can be achieved and memory can be improved.

Then again, stress can also hamper memory retrieval. In their experiments, the researchers have found that being exposed to stress prior to a memory retention test can result in poor performance.

How Poor Nutrition Negatively Affects the Brain

For decades, experts have proven that the food you eat directly affects your behavior and cognitive performance. For example, coffee can stimulate your brain while sugar can make children hyperactive. Chocolate can also make you feel good.

In the recent years, however, further studies have been made on the nutritional effects of food on the brain. In particular, researchers have discovered that certain types of food affect mood disorders, disease states, aging, cognition, and brain development.

A major effect of nutrition on brain function is on cognition. Poor diet can negatively affect energy levels, mood, and sleeping patterns. Also, cognition can be indirectly affected by other brain function developments. For example, nutrition is necessary to develop sensory systems such as vision and hearing. If these systems are not fully developed, cognitive maturation cannot be achieved.

Nutrition also directly affects cognition during neurodevelopment and aging. Getting the right nutrients is absolutely crucial during these times. Otherwise, the functioning of the brain cannot be optimized.

How Diet Affects Brain Function

At the Neuroscience 2012, the annual meeting of members of the Society for Neuroscience, it was found that the brain's biological processes can affect serious medical conditions, such as obesity and diabetes.

The researchers used imaging technologies to study the way neurology affects dietary disorders. They found that what people eat affects what and how they think.

They found that the cognitive function of an individual is influenced by obesity. This means that more efforts are necessary to complete a complex decision-making activity.

When you skip breakfast, the part of your brain associated with pleasure gets turned on after seeing images of food that are high in calories. Also, skipping breakfast can cause you to eat more at lunch.

In one study, it was found that a high-sugar diet can affect the insulin receptors of the brain as well as undermine memory and spatial learning skills. Nonetheless, this effect may be compensated by taking omega-3 supplements.

Fernando Gomez-Pinilla, a professor of neurosurgery and physiological science at the University of California, Los Angeles, said that food is akin to pharmaceutical compounds that affect the brain. Sleep, diet, and exercise can all affect your mental function and brain health. Hence, changing your diet can also enhance your cognitive skills, counteract the effects of aging, and protect your brain against damage.

The omega-3 fatty acids contained in walnuts, kiwi, and salmon are effective in improving memory and enhancing learning abilities. They can also reduce your risk of mental health problems such as mood disorders, dementia, depression, and schizophrenia.

Omega-3 fatty acids also support synaptic plasticity as well as positively influence the expression of molecules associated with memory and learning. These fatty acids are vital for normal brain development.

When you lack this nutrient, you can be at risk of attention-deficit disorder, dementia, bipolar disorder, schizophrenia, and dyslexia among other mental illnesses. It may also impair your memory and learning.

Coconut oil is another nutrient that is good for the brain. According to Dr. Mary Newport, a researcher, two tablespoons of coconut oil can provide you with twenty grams of medium-chain triglycerides, which can fight against degenerative neurological diseases.

Choline is also essential for your brain. It keeps the cell membranes in top shape and plays a significant role in nerve communications. It also prevents the accumulation of homocysteine in the blood and reduces the risk of chronic inflammation.

With proper diet, you can prevent brain injury and improve brain function.

Chapter 3: Apply Memorization Techniques to All Areas of Your Personal and Professional Life. Remember Names, Numbers, Lists, and Even Impress Your Friends

You have previously read about Ed Cooke, co-founder and CEO of Memrise, and his unusual expertise. According to his team, the following techniques can help you sharpen your memory:

Memrise Techniques

Be mindful of the location.

Context can mess with your memory severely. Say, you are in the kitchen when you suddenly thought of getting your coat from your bedroom. You go upstairs only to forget what you came there for. So, you head back downstairs and suddenly remember about the coat.

To prevent this from happening again, you should visualize what you are searching for in your chosen location. This way, your new context will hold the memory of what you need.

Train your brain.

Keep your brain active by acquiring new information constantly. You can read books, do crossword puzzles, learn a foreign language, and engage in intellectual conversations. See to it that your mind is always stimulated.

Play mind games.

Each memory is unique. Nevertheless, you can play certain games that are beneficial to the mind. For example, you can ask a friend to list down twenty words and ask you to reproduce them in exact order. Do your best to remember the words. Keep practicing until your brain becomes accustomed to this exercise.

Repeat.

As the saying goes, "repetition is key". Cooke conducted an online experiment that involved memory experts. They were asked to state the best techniques for memorization, and repetition was among their answers.

Words and simple concepts may have to be repeated up to thirty times before they stick. On the other hand, job presentations and speeches may require more repetitions since they are more complicated.

As much as possible, you should aim to comprehend the essence of whatever you are trying to memorize so that you can avoid making mistakes.

Tell a story.

The human brain is fond of stories. In fact, character-driven narratives can cause oxytocin to be released. This is the hormone that promotes empathy.

Stories have the characteristic of information that makes the brain remember and grow fond of it. This is why companies often use stories in their advertisements. They want people to remember their brands through the stories that they tell.

Other Effective Techniques You Can Use

The following are also highly recommended for improving your memory:

he Loci Technique

This ancient technique has been around for thousands of years. It originated in Ancient Greece and is also commonly referred to as "the memory palace".

In a study published in The American Physiological Society, it was found that 92.9% of the student participants were able to improve their information recall after three sixty-minute training sessions. The longer they practice the loci technique, the better their performance became.

The theory behind this technique is simple and straightforward. You must associate the things that you are trying to remember with specific images and places.

Ideally, you should choose a place with a personal significance, such as your bedroom or your favorite restaurant. This way, you will find the things inside them interesting and worth remembering.

The loci technique is effective in remembering information that has to be recalled but not processed, such as faces, names, lists, and birthdays.

Here is an example on how to use the loci technique or memory palace technique in everyday life:

1. Visualize yourself standing in your favorite place, such as your bedroom.

2. Mentally walk through your bedroom and notice any distinctive features that you can use to store the things that you want to remember. Every stop on your path would be a "loci". For instance, your bedroom door may be the first loci and your bed the second loci. Remember these features so that when you think of this location, the objects and route in it will be ingrained in your memory.

3. Associate the things that you have to recall with the loci in your favorite location or "palace". Say, you have a grocery list. You can imagine coffee flooding your bedroom door and oatmeal cookies on your bed. Instead of seeing a nightstand, you can imagine an apple in its place. This may seem absurd, but it can actually make you remember your grocery list.

nemonics

This technique is popular among elementary students. When you were little, you may have used it to remember the months of the year or the correct order of the planets. Does "My Very Educated Mother Just Served Us Nine Pizzas" ring a bell to you?

In 2017, a study was conducted at the University of Florida. The researchers evaluated the effectiveness of mnemonics and learned that 71.2% of the student participants found it to be helpful in remembering and understanding study materials better.

Musical Mnemonics

These mnemonics are highly effective, especially in helping people remember and retain academic content, because they provide structure for information as well as encourage repetition.

People generally find it easier to recall catchy songs and tunes than to remember long strings of letters or words. This is the main reason why companies and even politicians use jingles to promote themselves and make their brands or messages stick.

For example, schoolchildren are taught the alphabet using the ABC song. Older students also sing the period table song to memorize the elements.

Expression Mnemonics or Acronyms

Just like when you used "My Very Educated Mother Just Served Us Nine Pizzas" to memorize the plants, you also probably used "Every Good Boy Does Fine" to memorize the lines of the treble clef (EGBDF) in music.

Likewise, you can remember the expression "looks the same, cooks the same" to remember chopping and dicing ingredients uniformly to cook food evenly.

Rhyming Mnemonics

These are similar to musical mnemonics, except that the ending of every line should rhyme. They create a pattern that is easy to recall. For example, there is a rhyme that helps you remember how many days every month has.

hyming Peg System

It is also referred to as the hook system. It is often used to memorize lists of items. For every number, you have to memorize a picture of the word that rhymes with it. This will give you a peg or hook for the things that you have to remember in order.

For example, if you have a list of grocery items and you have to remember them in order, you can use the following peg system:

1. Create or learn your rhyming peg, such as one bun, two shoe, three tree, etc.

2. Create a clear picture of the rhyming object of every number. In this example, you can visualize a bread bun, a running shoe, and a pine tree. Pay attention to their details, such as the material of the shoe or the color of the leaves.

3. Imagine the rhyming object along with the item on your list. So, if your first item is hotdogs, you can imagine a hotdog sandwich. This is pretty simple since a hotdog in a bread bun is a pretty common sight. However, if your first item is milk, it can be quite ridiculous to imagine it being poured into a bread bun. Nonetheless, you should not hesitate to visualize these things, no matter how odd they may seem. You can visualize a milk container placed between bread buns. If your second item is chocolate chip cookies, you can imagine them being stored inside running shoes.

This technique requires quite a lot of creativity and effort. Nonetheless, it is very effective in helping people retain information longer as compared to when they try to merely memorize the words. Also, once you get used to your rhyming peg, you can use it for other lists in the future.

hunking

This technique involves grouping things together so that they can be recalled easier and faster. It is ideal for memorizing social security IDs, bank account numbers, and phone numbers.

Its key aspect is grouping items according to semantic encoding. This means that things should be placed in groups based on pattern or context. For example, you may group your grocery list according to type or brand. Find a pattern that you are comfortable with.

If you want to learn a foreign language, you can sort vocabulary words by topic. You can also arrange list items according to their first letters or how many letters they have. You can also associate things with the larger group that they may belong to. For example, you can remember pizza = crust, cheese, sauce, pepperoni.

When it comes to memorizing numbers, such as phone numbers, you may group similar numbers together. For example, you can remember "000" "555" "7777" instead of "0005557777".

According to studies, the human brain is capable of holding four different things in its short-term or working memory. When you group data into smaller groups, you may hack the limits of your short-term or working memory so that you can remember more information.

This technique is effective because the human brain is designed to search for patterns and form connections.

he Building Technique

It may be built over the other techniques. It can also help people remember more data aside from simple facts, phone numbers, and names.

It is true that remembering facts is helpful. However, you need to have a profound understanding and deep knowledge of your profession or field of study as well.

A concept or fact that is fully understood has a greater chance of retaining in memory than something that is merely memorized. When you introduce meaning or a sense of understanding to the things that you want to remember, you can remember them better as well as apply them in various contexts.

ind Maps

They are highly beneficial in improving creative thinking. However, they can also be used to learn new information and organize them more coherently.

A mind map has the elements of the building technique and the loci technique. It is effective in organizing huge, complex subjects into visual categories that are distinguishable. It can also break down multiple documents or long texts.

For example, if you just got hired, you can use mind maps to understand the products and/or services that your company offers. You can also use this technique to create your own marketing and sales strategies.

You can find software programs for mind mapping online. However, you can also create your own. For example, you can use a pen and paper. Simply write down an idea or topic that you want to remember. Express it using one to two words. Then, you should connect it to sub-topics according to relevance.

Lifestyle Modifications and Improvements

Of course, your diet, exercise routine, and general lifestyle play a huge role in your mental wellness. A healthy lifestyle brings about positive long-term effects on memory.

Hence, you should ensure that you get sufficient amounts of rest and sleep. You should also exercise on a regular basis and have a balanced diet. Start moving around if you have always been sedentary. Physical movements enhance learning skills and protect the memory.

Researchers at Harvard Medical School conducted a study in which the participants did an hour of brisk walking twice a week for six months. After the study, it was found that the hippocampus of the participants increased in size. This is the area of the brain that is associated with learning and verbal memory.

According to the researchers, it is crucial to do challenging exercises to elevate the pulse. This increases blood flow to the brain and ensures that enough oxygen is transported.

Dormancy is also crucial for a good memory. Researchers from Germany and Boston conducted a study that showed how lack of sleep affects the ability to perform simple tasks such as name recall and face recognition.

The participants were divided into two groups. The ones that stayed awake all night performed poorly compared to the participants that slept for eight hours before doing their tasks. This proves that sleep is necessary for optimum brain function.

The brain resets during sleep. It clears out neuron build up at nighttime to let you wake up refreshed and relaxed.

A balanced diet is also necessary. As you know, what you eat can affect the way you think, talk, and behave. For example, foods that are high in cholesterol can cause heart diseases. Such cholesterol can also build up in the brain, causing blood flow restriction and insufficient oxygen supply.

Time Blocking and Stuff Offloading

To keep your brain healthy, you need to take a break once in a while. Rather than try to remember everything, you can automate certain tasks or data such as birthdays, to-do lists, and shopping lists.

You can use time blocking, which is about blocking off time on a calendar to allow the brain to quit thinking about tasks since the time to do them has already been allocated. This helps the brain concentrate on tasks that are much more important. See to it that you also track how much time you spend doing your tasks so that you can properly adjust your blocks.

The human brain is amazing. Neurons are able to store multiple memories at once. Your mental capacity is around 2.5 petabytes. Nonetheless, even though it is highly unlikely for your brain to get full, it is still much better for you to offload certain information to digital tools.

For example, you can use Evernote to create to-do lists and manage your tasks. Apps like this are effective in increasing productivity. You can find a variety of other similar tools online. Download and use the ones that best fit your needs.

The above mentioned techniques are highly recommended by scientists. Although there are still a lot of mysteries that surround the human brain, these techniques will surely help you sharpen your memory and attain your goals.

Chapter 4: By Memorizing a Pack of Playing Cards

Is it possible to memorize a deck of playing cards in less than a minute? This may sound absurd, but the answer to this question is an astounding 'yes'. Even if you do not have a photographic memory, you can train yourself to have it.

Ed Cooke was, in fact, the Grand Master of Memory. When he was twenty-three years old, he memorized the order of ten decks of cards in sixty minutes and a shuffled deck of cards in just forty-three seconds. He also memorized one thousand random digits in sixty minutes and the order of a deck of cards in less than a couple of minutes.

Even better, he helped Joshua Foer, a journalist, to become Memory Champion in just one year. Foer memorized 120 random digits in five minutes as well as a shuffled deck of cards in over a minute. He also memorized the names of more than one hundred strangers in fifteen minutes.

What can you get from memorizing a deck of playing cards, you say? Aside from sharpening your memory and impressing a ton of people, you also get the chance to win thousands of dollars in competitions. This is a pretty good deal.

The Bicycleshop

This is the method Cooke used to memorize the playing cards. It is a combination of Photoshop and the playing card brand. It has two versions: Bicycleshop Lite and Bicycleshop Pro.

icycleshop Lite

It lets you memorize the playing cards as well as their order.

Step 1: Learn the cards.

You need to convert the fifty-two playing cards into fifty-two celebrities. As you know, the human brain does not remember the mundane. So, you need to give it something unusual in order for the information to stick.

As much as possible, you should attach a personality type and a profession to every card. This way, you will have two cues for every celebrity. Here is an example:

Spade cards – weird or amusing individuals

Club cards – tough individuals

Heart cards – lovable individuals

Diamond cards – wealthy individuals

The Playing Cards

You can associate these cards with professions. Odd numbers can be male while even numbers can be female. Pair up these cards. Then, remember that they represent powerful individuals. For example, 10's are powerful women while 9's are powerful men.

In order to facilitate such association, you have to include mnemonics below every profession. For example, the Queen can be the female half of celebrity couples while the King is the male half. This is relevant since celebrity couples are treated like royalty, anyway.

Jacks can represent religious figures and bachelors. 10 and 9 are the highest numbers. So, it is only fitting that they are used to represent the highest-powered individuals.

8s can be popular female physiques and 7s can be popular male physiques. Think of ripped or busty individuals. 6s can be controversial females while 5s are controversial males. After all, the number six sounds a lot like the word sex.

4s can be movie actresses and 3s can be movie actors. You can think of the movie trilogies. Finally, 2s can be female athletes and aces can be male athletes. Ace is often associated with sports excellence. You can also think of 2 as the "deuce" used in tennis.

Putting Everything Together

Now that you have selected four personalities and thirteen professions, you already have seventeen things to remember. You can use your current opinions and knowledge to fill in your 52-card matrix.

For example, you can think of the ace of diamonds as a man who became rich. Ace is associated with men while diamonds are associated with wealth. Your ace of diamonds can be Michael Jordan.

Then, the jack of spades can be an amusing religious figure. This can be the Dalai Lama, who is humorous and clever. The six of spades can be a controversial woman, such as Lady Gaga.

Through this method, you can fill out your matrix in less than one hour and successfully remember the individuals that represent the fifty-two playing cards. You can also shuffle your deck of cards and translate them to their images. Do not stop until everything sticks to your memory and becomes automatic. It may take an hour for you to do this. When you are done, you can arrange them in order.

Step 2: Memorize the order of the shuffled deck of cards.

You can now peg fifty-two cards to familiar locations. This can be a path from your driveway to your favorite café or a short distance from your bedroom to the garden. Choose whatever feels comfortable for you.

Some memory experts visualize their childhood homes. For instance, Scott Hogwood, U.S. Memory Champion from 2001 to 2004, used rooms from Architectural Digest luxury homes. When you use this method, you may position yourself mentally at the front door of every room. Then, you can move from where you are to the left and right corners, and eventually to the ceiling.

It only takes half an hour to select fifty-two locations. Then, you may begin positioning the celebrities at every point. At first, you can keep things simple. As you go on, you can use longer and more complicated paths.

So, for example, you can think of the Dalai Lama as the Jack of Spades. Visualize him standing at your front door, which is your first point. Then, visualize him at your second point, and so on.

Pay close attention to the details of the images in your head. Once you reach the end of your route, you should trace it back in your imagination. You should be able to remember every individual in your imagined sequence. You may have to go over this sequence two to three times before it sticks to your memory.

icycleshop Pro

This is an upgraded version of the Bicycleshop Lite. It is ideal for people who want to use a more effective compression algorithm. This method builds on top of the things that you already know.

With Bicycleshop Lite, you used fifty-two images. With this version, you can simply use seventeen to eighteen images so that you can memorize things much faster.

Still using the celebrities you assigned to the cards, you can associate them with a particular object and action.

For example, you can visualize the Dalai Lama praying and Michael Jordan playing basketball. The object associated with the Dalai Lama is the Buddha while the action associated with him is praying. The object associated with Michael Jordan is basketball while the action associated with him is dunking.

When you add this syntactic structure, your combination of cards can form short sentences that involve the celebrity from the first card, the action from the second card, and the object from the third card.

Using these methods require time and effort. You have to practice them several times until you get used to them. Don't worry because your efforts will not turn out to be futile. These methods are guaranteed to help you remember and memorize various things.

Chapter 5: Discover the Secret of the Oldest Memory Trick that Dates Back to Around 500 B.C.

You have read about the Loci Method, also referred to as the Method of Loci, in a previous chapter. This memory improvement technique is actually the oldest, dating back to the days of the Roman Empire.

The Method of Loci

"Loci," a word that is actually the plural of locus, refers to place or location. So, this technique is founded on the supposition that familiar places are the easiest to remember. When you associate something with a location or place that you know by heart, you can use this location or place as your clue to recall the information.

The loci method is a unique linking strategy. Simonides of Ceos, a poet who became the sole survivor of a tragedy, developed this method as attributed by Cicero.

Ceos was attending a banquet in Thessaly with several other people when their building collapsed. Although it was hard to identify the victims due to their conditions, he identified them by recalling where they were seated. This experience made him realize that it is possible to recall anything simply by correlating it with mental images of placements.

Greek and Roman orators also used this method to give public speeches without using notes. This technique gained intense popularity from 500 B.C. to the mid-1600s. It is best for people who have excellent visualizing skills.

How to Use the Method of Loci

Here are the steps on how to use this ancient method of remembering information:

Step 1: Picture a location or place that you know really well.

This can be anywhere, such as your home or office. Visualize certain paths in this location in a logical manner.

For example, you can visualize the route that you usually take to go from your bedroom to your backyard. Start at your bedroom door, walk down the hall, head to the kitchen, get out of the back door, and finally go to the backyard.

As you go through each location, you have to move consistently and logically in a single direction. You can also consider appliances and furniture pieces as additional locations.

Step 2: Put every object that you want to recall in every location.

Whenever you want to remember these things, you can simply imagine your home and go to every room in it. Every object that you associated a certain place inside your home must come into your mind as you imagine yourself going to each and every one of these places.

Say, you want to remember these items on your grocery list: toothpaste, deodorant, mustard, bread, and eggs.

As you imagine your home, you should also imagine toothpaste all over your front door. Do not just visualize the word "toothpaste". You have to really see the object in your mind. Imagine yourself pressing the tube and letting the toothpaste squeeze out of it. Recall the taste, smell, and feel of the toothpaste too.

Next, imagine yourself entering through the front door and walking down the hall to see a huge deodorant walking towards you. Imagine yourself walking past it to go to the living room. Here, you see a tall bottle of mustard dancing. Its yellow color is so bright; it's almost blinding.

You go to the kitchen to see a bread bun sitting while it stares at a fat egg wearing an apron. It goes to a frying pan to crack and cook itself.

Once you have visually positioned every item around your home, it would be easier for you to recall your grocery list. Simply imagine your front door. Your subconscious mind will immediately associate it with the toothpaste. Then, imagine your hallway to remember deodorant, and so on.

Do not hesitate to unleash your creativity. Be as outrageous as you can. The more interesting and absurd your mental pictures are, the easier it would be for you to recall them accurately.

The method of loci is not only effective in helping you remember lists. It is also useful in remembering important parts of speeches, names of people, tasks you have to do, and ideas that you want to share or turn into a project.

This method is very effective because it alters the way the mind remembers things. It involves the use of familiar places to give you cues about specific things. Since these places are organized in a manner that you are familiar with, every memory flows smoothly to the next.

You may also adapt this method by including buildings and other structures that you are familiar with. For example, you can visualize a church, mall, your best friend's house, etc.

It does not really matter how far or close apart every place is. The only thing that matters is how distinct they are from one another. With this being said, you may want to avoid picturing the library in your mind since it has identical aisles and shelves, and this might only confuse you. The places you visualize should be unique, memorable, and distinct.

You may also put several items in one location. For example, if you have fifty items on your grocery list, you can imagine five items in one location and another set of five items in the next location, and so on.

The Method of Loci In Modern Times

Although ancient, the method of loci is still useful today. In fact, it is widely used in contemporary memory competitions, such as the United States Memory Championship and the World Memory Championship. These competitions require memorizing sequences of numbers, letters, and playing cards.

Some of the most notable individuals who used the method of loci include Dominic O'Brien, Clemens Mayer, and Simon Reinhard. This technique is also taught as a metacognitive strategy in learning-to-learn courses. It is used to encode the main ideas of a particular subject.

Chapter 6: Powerful Memory Techniques and Memory Skills to Increase Brain Function

By now, you should already know that brain health is significantly affected by diet and lifestyle. Aside from using accelerated learning techniques, you should also get adequate nutrition.

The way you eat and behave contributes to your cognitive decline. Hence, you should ensure that you get sufficient amounts of rest and sleep, a balanced diet, and a stress-free environment.

Moreover, a healthy lifestyle supports brain health and promotes neurogenesis or the process that involves growing new neurons. The hippocampus or the memory center of the brain is capable of producing new cells. It actually regenerates your whole life. So, even in your old age, your brain can still produce new neurons, as long as you keep it in top shape.

The following are some of the things you can do to learn faster, improve your brain function, and keep your brain healthy:

Exercise

You know how important exercise is. It stimulates the nerve cells to multiply so that your brain can work at its optimum capacity. It also strengthens the interconnections of nerve cells as well as protects them against damage.

When you exercise, your nerve cells release neurotrophic factors, which are proteins. The brain-derived neurotrophic factor triggers chemicals that lead to neural health.

In 2010, a study on primates was published in Neuroscience. It showed that regular exercise improves blood flow to the brain and promotes learning. These findings are also applicable to humans. In another study, it was found that those who exercised on a regular basis were able to grow and expand their memory center up to two percent annually.

Get Enough Sleep

According to researchers at Harvard University, people are thirty-three percent more likely to deduce connections among ideas that are not closely related after they have slept. However, only a few of them notice the improvements in their performance.

Sleep can enhance your memory. It can also help you practice your skills in order to improve them further. Simply getting four to six hours of sleep is already enough to influence your abilities to think clearly.

Neuroplasticity is said to underlie the capacity of the brain to manage behaviors, including memory and learning. Plasticity happens when the neurons get stimulated by information or events from external sources. Nonetheless, sleep loss and sleep alter the expressions of certain genes that might be necessary for synaptic plasticity.

In addition, some types of long term potentiation that are connected to the laying down of memory and learning may be elicited in sleep. This suggests that synaptic connections get stronger when you sleep. Even an afternoon nap can significantly restore and boost your brainpower.

Play Brain Games

When you do not challenge your brain, it starts to deteriorate. So, in order to keep your brain in top shape, you have to provide it with the right stimulus. For instance, you can play brain games.

There are lots of games available for brain training, particularly on the Internet. Websites such as Lumosity.com, for example, is a great source. Brain HQ is another ideal website with various brain exercises. They allow users to monitor and track their progress.

Dr. Michael Merzenich, a professor at the University of California, pioneered brain plasticity research. He also created a computer-based program to train the brain.

This can sharpen your skills, from memorization to reading and comprehension.

Ideally, you should spend at least twenty minutes per day on brain games but you should not spend more than seven minutes on one task. The benefits of brain games tend to weaken when they are overdone.

Dr. Merzenich said that primary benefits are observed within the first six minutes of performing the task. Then again, if you are too busy, playing brain games may seem like an additional task rather than a new hobby.

Master New Skills

The neurological system gets stimulated when you engage in meaningful and purposeful activities. Likewise, these activities also counter the effects of diseases that are related to stress as well as reduce the risk of dementia. Choose tasks that attract your attention in order for them to be effective in boosting your brain health.

In one study, it was found that quilting, knitting, and other craft activities were connected to reduced chances of experiencing mild cognitive impairment. In another study, it was found that engaging in cognitively demanding activities such as taking digital photography improved the memory of older adults.

This technique would only be effective when you choose activities that stimulate you mentally. They should require your undivided attention as well as give you satisfaction. They should be activities that you are excited to do, such as painting, gardening, etc.

Intermittent Fasting

Ketones, not glucose, are fuel for the brain. They are fats that get mobilized by the body when carbohydrates are no longer consumed. This is why you have to consume healthy fats such as coconut oil.

Fasting for one day is enough to reset itself and burn fats instead of sugar. Moreover, it can reduce your total consumption of calories. This can promote the growth of brain cells.

As much as possible, you should restrict your eating schedule to a six- to eight-hour window. This would allow you to fast for sixteen to eighteen hours per day.

Chapter 7: Protect Your Memory from Deteriorating Due to the Aging Process

When you reach fifty years of age, you may notice certain changes in your body, including a decline in memory. Although memory lapses may occur at any age, they tend to occur more often with aging. They are typically caused by neurological illness, brain injuries, and organic disorders.

According to researchers, you may reduce your risk of dementia and prevent cognitive decline by living a healthy lifestyle. They especially recommend the Mediterranean diet, which involves vegetables, fruits, healthy fats, and whole grains.

Dr. Argye Hillis, a neurology professor at John Hopkins Medicine, said that you should refrain from eating red meats. In one study, it was found that those who followed this diet were twenty percent less likely to develop memory and thinking problems.

Most memory problems reflect natural brain changes, which may slow down the cognitive process and make it more difficult for you to process new information. Fortunately, there are a lot of things you can do to protect your memory from deteriorating.

Get treatment for pre-existing conditions.

Most of the medical issues that impair cognitive abilities are untreated or unrecognized. Hence, you need to get regular checkups to ensure that you are in excellent health. In case you get diagnosed with an illness, see to it that you have it treated right away.

For example, if you have diabetes, you have to follow your doctor's orders to treat your condition. Blood surges can hamper your memory by decreasing the supply of blood to your brain.

You should also manage your blood pressure since memory lapses can be caused by hypertension. In a study published in Neurology in 2009, it was found that the rate of memory issues increased by seven percent for every ten-point rise in diastolic blood pressure.

Researchers have also found that individuals with sleep apnea tend to score worse on cognitive and memory tests. However, when they keep their airways open as they sleep, they are able to get better scores.

Moreover, cognitive problems may be symptoms of depression. Women are especially prone to this mental problem. Their skills tend to decline quickly and they become more prone to developing Alzheimer's disease.

Don't forget to have your thyroid levels checked. Take note that hypothyroidism may affect memory, attention, and learning. With proper treatment, a better cognitive performance can be achieved.

You should also watch your cholesterol levels. High cholesterol levels can increase your risk of Alzheimer's disease and cognitive impairment. In a 2008 study, it was found that memory decline and low HDL levels are related to each other.

Take a memory course.

As much as possible, you should take a memory course that is run by experts in cognitive rehabilitation or psychology. See to it that it also focuses on the practical methods of managing daily challenges. Avoid courses that focus on concentration or computer games since they are not very helpful in real-world scenarios.

Keep your social life active.

Book clubs and other organizations are great because they keep you socially connected to other people. This helps your brain stay active. The more connections you have, the better you can preserve your memory and mental function.

Additionally, social interactions can boost your mood. This can help you prevent depression, which is a common cause of dementia.

Manage stress properly.

Stressors will always be around. You cannot magically make stress disappear from your life. As you grow, you encounter people, situations, and other factors that can make you stressed. When your body releases too much cortisol, you may find it hard to recall information.

This is why you should find time to relax and refresh once in a while. You can go to a spa and get a massage. You can also soak yourself in a hot tub. You can also try yoga and meditation. Whatever you do, make sure that it relaxes your mind and body.

Use memory tactics.

Each time you learn a new word or name, you can repeat it loudly so that it gets stuck in your memory. You can also mentally connect new words or names with images. For example, if you get introduced to someone named June, you can imagine a woman in a wedding dress to represent the month of June. You can also post sticky notes all over your office and home. You can also set reminders on your phone as well as mark your calendars to remember vital details.

Conclusion

I'd like to thank you and congratulate you for transiting my lines from start to finish.

I hope this book was able to help you learn about the different strategies you can use to improve your memory.

Having a sharp memory is beneficial to the different aspects of your life, including your personal relationships, health, finances, business, and career. It will not only impress your family members and friends, but it will also keep your brain in top shape.

In addition, it will prevent you from being embarrassed during social gatherings when you see someone you know by face but has forgotten their name. Having a sharp memory can also save your life since you can avoid making the same mistakes.

This book is all about sharpening the memory in order to learn faster and be more productive. It also discusses how certain factors, such as poor nutrition, can directly affect the brain.

It is also about training the brain to develop a long-term working memory. It will teach you how to remember lists, series of numbers, names, and even a deck of playing cards. Moreover, it is about conditioning yourself to become a memory master as well as to keep your brain healthy even in old age.

I hope that you follow the tips and recommendations stated in this book. Not everyone has a sharp memory. You are fortunate to find this book and get a chance to improve your memory.

The next step is to apply the lessons that you have learned into your life.

I wish you the best of luck!

Thanks for Reading

What did you think of, **Limitless: Master the Art of Memory Improvement with Brain Training to Learn Faster, Remember More, Increase Productivity and Improve Memory**

I know you could have picked any number of books to read, but you picked this book and for that I am extremely grateful.

I hope that it added at value and quality to your everyday life. If so, it would be really nice if you could share this book with your friends and family by posting to [Facebook](#) and [Twitter](#).

If you enjoyed this book and found some benefit in reading this, I'd like to hear from you and hope that you could take some time to post a review. Your feedback and support will help this author to greatly improve his writing craft for future projects and make this book even better.

I want you, the reader, to know that your review is very important and so, if you'd like to leave a review, all you have to do is click here and away you go. I wish you all the best in your future success!

Thank you and good luck

Trustgenics

Claim your FREE Audiobook Now

The Confident New You - Develop Your Confidence and Start Living the Life You Deserve

Do you get lost for words around other people, or do you suffer from social anxiety? Are you more concerned about how you look to other people?

If your confidence is always holding you back from achieving what you really want in your life, or if you have always been super shy with no confidence then read on.

You're about to discover how to be confident in any situation. Find out how to make a great first impression and keep the conversation going, without appearing awkward.

Learn to stop thinking negatively about yourself and conquer your fears to gain unstoppable confidence at anything. Even if you don't have low confidence, you can always benefit from improved confidence - there are always greater heights to reach.

THE CONFIDENT NEW YOU

DEVELOP YOUR CONFIDENCE AND START LIVING THE LIFE YOU DESERVE

DARCY CARTER

Trustgenics

Master key ideas in math, science, and computer science through problem solving.

Sign up for Free Now

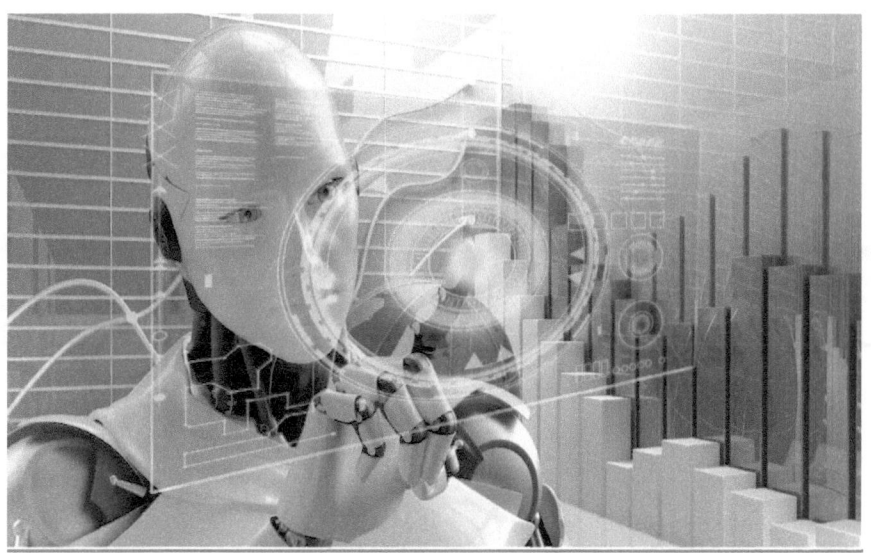

www.ingramcontent.com/pod-product-compliance
Lightning Source LLC
Chambersburg PA
CBHW021124080526
44587CB00010B/624